BREAKIN ESTROGEN

A Guide To Understanding Imbalances, Impact On Women's Health, How To Overcome Hormonal Imbalances And Regain Your Vitality.

By

Dr. Karen Jones

Copyright©2023 Dr.KarenJones

All Rights Reserved

TABLE OF CONTENT

INTRODUCTION

CHAPTER 1 - The Importance Of Hormonal Balance: An Introduction To Estrogen Imbalance

CHAPTER 2 - Understanding Estrogen: The Role Of Hormones In Women's Health.

CHAPTER 3 - Estrogen Imbalance: Causes And Risk Factors

CHAPTER 4 - Signs And Symptoms Of Estrogen Imbalance: How To Recognize Hormonal Disruption

CHAPTER 5 - Diagnostic Testing For Estrogen Imbalance: Methods And Limitations

CHAPTER 6 - Treating Estrogen Imbalance: Lifestyle Changes, Medications, And Alternative Therapies

CHAPTER 7 - Managing Menopause - Addressing Estrogen Imbalance and Aging

CHAPTER 8 - Estrogen And Women's Health: The Link To Breast Cancer, Heart Disease, And Other Conditions

CHAPTER 9 - Balancing Estrogen Naturally: Strategies for Optimal Hormonal Health

CHAPTER 10 - Living With Estrogen Imbalance: Coping With The Emotional And Physical Challenges

CONCLUSION

INTRODUCTION

Hormones are the body's chemical messengers that regulate various bodily functions, including growth and development, metabolism, reproduction, and mood. One of the key hormones in a woman's body is estrogen, which plays a crucial role in reproductive health, bone density, heart health, and cognitive function.

However, when the hormonal balance is disrupted, it can lead to a range of health problems, including estrogen imbalance. Estrogen imbalance occurs when there is either too much or too little estrogen in the body. This imbalance can have a significant impact on a woman's health, leading to various physical and emotional symptoms.

In this book, "Breaking the Estrogen Cycle," we will delve into the topic of estrogen imbalance and its impact on women's health. We will explore the various causes and risk factors of estrogen imbalance, how to recognize the signs and symptoms of hormonal disruption, and diagnostic testing methods.

We will also discuss the treatment options available to women who are struggling with estrogen imbalance. This includes lifestyle changes, medications, and alternative therapies, as well as natural strategies for optimal hormonal health.

In addition, we will explore the impact of estrogen imbalance on women's health, including the link between estrogen and breast cancer, heart disease, and other conditions. We will discuss the ways in which women can take control of their health and regain their vitality by breaking the estrogen cycle.

This book is designed to provide women with a comprehensive guide to understanding estrogen imbalance and how it impacts their health. It offers practical advice and strategies for overcoming hormonal imbalances, improving overall health, and regaining vitality.

Whether you are struggling with hormonal imbalances or simply want to learn more about how to optimize your hormonal health, Breaking the Estrogen Cycle is the ultimate guide for women looking to take control of their health and live their best lives.

CHAPTER 1

The Importance Of Hormonal Balance: An Introduction To Estrogen Imbalance

Our overall health and well-being are significantly impacted by hormones.
They are responsible for regulating several bodily functions such as growth, metabolism, sexual development, and reproduction. Hormonal balance is essential to maintaining optimal health, but when there is an imbalance, it can lead to several health problems, including estrogen imbalance.

Estrogen is a hormone that is primarily produced in the ovaries in women and in small amounts in men's testes. It is responsible for developing and maintaining female sexual characteristics, such as breast development, regulation of the menstrual cycle, and bone density. However, an imbalance in estrogen levels can lead to a wide range of health issues.

Estrogen imbalance can occur due to several reasons, including age, genetics, lifestyle factors, and medical conditions. In this article, we will discuss the importance of hormonal balance and the causes and symptoms of estrogen imbalance.

The Importance Of Hormonal Balance

Hormonal balance is crucial to our overall health and well-being. Hormones act as chemical messengers in our body, communicating with various organs and tissues and regulating their functions. When hormones are in balance, our body functions optimally, and we feel healthy and energetic.

However, when there is an imbalance in hormone levels, it can lead to several health problems. For instance, an imbalance in estrogen levels can lead to weight gain, mood swings, irregular periods, decreased sex drive, and even an increased risk of certain cancers, such as breast cancer.

Estrogen Imbalance: Causes And Symptoms

Estrogen imbalance can occur due to several reasons, including age, genetics, lifestyle factors, and medical conditions. Let's take a look at some of the common causes of estrogen imbalance:

Age: As women age, their estrogen levels decline. This decline usually occurs during menopause, which is the time when a woman stops having periods. During menopause, the ovaries stop producing estrogen, and the body's estrogen levels decline significantly.

Genetics: Some women may be predisposed to estrogen imbalance due to their genetics. For instance, women with a family history of breast cancer or other hormonal disorders may be at a higher risk of developing estrogen imbalance.

Lifestyle Factors: Certain lifestyle factors, such as a poor diet, lack of exercise, stress, and exposure to environmental toxins, can also contribute to estrogen imbalance.

Medical Conditions: Certain medical conditions, such as polycystic ovary syndrome (PCOS), thyroid disorders, and obesity, can also lead to estrogen imbalance.

Now that we know the common causes of estrogen imbalance, let's take a look at some of the symptoms:

Irregular Periods: Estrogen plays a crucial role in regulating the menstrual cycle. An imbalance in estrogen levels can lead to irregular periods, heavy bleeding, or no periods at all.

Weight Gain: Estrogen imbalance can lead to weight gain, particularly around the belly.

Mood Swings: Estrogen plays a crucial role in regulating mood. An imbalance in estrogen levels can lead to mood swings, irritability, and depression.

Decreased Sex Drive: Estrogen is responsible for regulating sex drive in women. An imbalance in estrogen levels can lead to a decreased sex drive.

Hot Flashes: Estrogen imbalance can lead to hot flashes, which are sudden feelings of warmth or heat that are often accompanied by sweating.

Breast Tenderness: Estrogen plays a crucial role in breast development. An imbalance in estrogen levels can lead to breast tenderness or swelling.

Fatigue: Estrogen plays a crucial role in regulating energy levels. An imbalance in estrogen levels can lead to fatigue or low energy levels.

CHAPTER 2

Understanding Estrogen: The Role Of Hormones In Women's Health.

Estrogen is one of the primary sex hormones in the female body, produced mainly by the ovaries, but also by the adrenal glands and fat cells. Estrogen levels fluctuate throughout a woman's life, affecting various bodily functions such as menstruation, bone density, and mood. This article will explore the role of estrogen in women's health, its effects on the body, and how estrogen levels change over time.

Functions Of Estrogen

Estrogen has numerous functions in the female body. The hormone is involved in the development of secondary sexual characteristics such as breast growth, pubic hair, and fat distribution. Estrogen also plays a vital role in reproductive health, regulating the menstrual cycle, ovulation, and pregnancy. The hormone also helps maintain vaginal health, promoting the growth of beneficial bacteria while keeping harmful bacteria at bay.

Estrogen also has an impact on bone health. It helps maintain bone density, preventing osteoporosis, a condition that weakens bones and makes them more prone to fracture. In addition, estrogen plays a role in the metabolism of fats, regulating cholesterol levels and reducing the risk of heart disease.

Estrogen And Menstrual Cycle
Regulating the menstrual cycle is significantly influenced by estrogen. The menstrual cycle is a complex process that involves the interplay of hormones, including estrogen, progesterone, and follicle-stimulating hormone (FSH). During the menstrual cycle, estrogen levels rise, causing the lining of the uterus to thicken, preparing it for implantation. When ovulation occurs, estrogen

levels peak, triggering the release of an egg from the ovary. If the egg is fertilized, estrogen levels remain high, supporting the pregnancy. If the egg is not fertilized, estrogen levels drop, and the menstrual cycle begins.

Estrogen Levels And Menopause

As women age, estrogen levels begin to decline. This decline is a natural part of the aging process and is often referred to as menopause. Menopause typically occurs between the ages of 45 and 55, with the average age being 51. During menopause, estrogen levels can fluctuate widely, leading to a range of symptoms such as hot flashes, night sweats, and vaginal dryness.

The decline in estrogen levels also has a significant impact on bone health. Without adequate estrogen levels, bones become more porous and prone to fractures, leading to osteoporosis. Women are at a higher risk of developing osteoporosis after menopause, and the risk increases with age.

Estrogen Therapy

Estrogen therapy is a medical treatment that involves the use of synthetic estrogen to replace the hormone that the body is no longer producing. Estrogen therapy can be delivered in various forms, including pills, patches, creams, and vaginal rings.

Estrogen therapy can help alleviate the symptoms of menopause, such as hot flashes and vaginal dryness. Reducing the risk of heart disease and preventing osteoporosis are additional benefits it may provide. However, estrogen therapy is not without risks. Women who undergo estrogen therapy may be at an increased risk of blood clots, stroke, and breast cancer. Therefore, it is essential to discuss the potential risks and benefits of estrogen therapy with a healthcare provider before undergoing treatment.

Estrogen And Breast Cancer

Research has established a correlation between estrogen and a heightened likelihood of developing breast cancer. Breast cancer arises in the breast cells, constituting a form of cancer. It is the most common cancer among women worldwide, accounting for 25% of all cancer cases in women.

Estrogen plays a role in the development and growth of some types of breast cancer. Women who have high levels of estrogen are at an increased risk of developing breast cancer. Women who undergo long-term estrogen therapy may also be at an increased risk of breast cancer.

CHAPTER 3

Estrogen Imbalance: Causes And Risk Factors

Estrogen is a hormone that plays a crucial role in a woman's reproductive system. It helps regulate the menstrual cycle, maintain bone density, and support cardiovascular health. Estrogen is produced primarily in the ovaries, but small amounts are also produced in the adrenal glands and fat tissues.

An estrogen imbalance occurs when there is too much or too little estrogen in the body.
A range of symptoms and health issues may arise as a result of this. Let us discuss the causes and risk factors of estrogen imbalance.

Causes Of Estrogen Imbalance
Menopause

Menopause is a natural part of a woman's life and occurs when the ovaries stop producing eggs. As a result, estrogen levels drop, and women may experience symptoms such as hot flashes, vaginal dryness, and mood swings.

On average, menopause tends to occur between the ages of 45 and 55.

Hormonal Birth Control

Hormonal birth control methods, such as the pill, patch, or ring, work by suppressing ovulation and preventing pregnancy. These methods contain synthetic hormones that mimic the effects of estrogen and progesterone. While they can be effective, they can also disrupt the body's natural hormone balance and lead to symptoms such as weight gain, mood changes, and decreased libido.

Polycystic Ovary Syndrome (PCOS)

PCOS, which stands for Polycystic Ovary Syndrome, is a condition characterized by hormonal imbalances that typically occur in women of reproductive age. It is characterized by the presence of multiple cysts on the ovaries, which can lead to irregular menstrual cycles and an overproduction of androgens (male hormones). This can cause a decrease in estrogen levels and lead to symptoms such as acne, weight gain, and excess hair growth.

Obesity

Fat tissue produces estrogen, so women who are overweight or obese may have higher levels of estrogen than women of normal weight. This can disrupt the body's natural hormone balance and lead to symptoms such as irregular menstrual cycles, breast tenderness, and mood swings.

Certain Medications

Certain medications, such as tamoxifen (used to treat breast cancer) and aromatase inhibitors (used to treat postmenopausal women with breast cancer), can interfere with estrogen production and lead to an estrogen imbalance.

Risk Factors For Estrogen Imbalance

Age

As women age, their estrogen levels naturally decline. This can lead to symptoms such as hot flashes, vaginal dryness, and mood changes.

Family History

A family history of estrogen-related disorders, such as breast cancer or ovarian cancer, can increase a woman's risk of developing an estrogen imbalance.

Menstrual Irregularities
Women who experience irregular menstrual cycles may be at an increased risk of developing an estrogen imbalance.

Stress
Stress can disrupt the body's natural hormone balance and lead to an estrogen imbalance.

Certain Health Conditions
Certain health conditions, such as thyroid disorders and autoimmune diseases, can disrupt the body's natural hormone balance and lead to an estrogen imbalance.

Symptoms Of Estrogen Imbalance

The symptoms of an estrogen imbalance can vary depending on whether there is too much or too little estrogen in the body. Some common symptoms of an estrogen imbalance include:

Irregular menstrual cycles
Hot flashes

Vaginal dryness
Mood swings
Decreased libido
Breast tenderness
Fatigue
Weight gain
Acne
Excess hair growth
Treatment for Estrogen Imbalance

The treatment for an estrogen imbalance will depend on the underlying cause and the severity of symptoms. Some common treatments include:

Hormone Replacement Therapy (HRT)
HRT is a common treatment for women going through menopause. Hormone replacement therapy entails administering estrogen and/or progesterone to compensate for the hormones that the body is not generating anymore. This can help alleviate symptoms such as hot flashes, vaginal dryness, and mood swings.

Birth Control Pills

Birth control pills can be used to regulate menstrual cycles and balance hormone levels. They contain synthetic versions of estrogen and progesterone, which can help to regulate the menstrual cycle and alleviate symptoms.

Lifestyle Changes
Making lifestyle changes such as maintaining a healthy weight, exercising regularly, and reducing stress can help to regulate hormone levels and alleviate symptoms.

Medications
Certain medications, such as anti-depressants and anti-anxiety medications, can be used to alleviate symptoms of an estrogen imbalance.

Surgery
In some cases, surgery may be necessary to treat an estrogen imbalance. For example, if a woman has an estrogen-producing tumor, surgery may be necessary to remove it.

Prevention Of Estrogen Imbalance

There are several steps that women can take to help prevent an estrogen imbalance:

Maintain A Healthy Weight
Maintaining a healthy weight can help to regulate hormone levels and prevent an estrogen imbalance.

Exercise Regularly
Regular exercise can help to regulate hormone levels and reduce stress, which can help to prevent an estrogen imbalance.

Eat A Healthy Diet
Eating a healthy diet that is rich in fruits, vegetables, whole grains, and lean protein can help to regulate hormone levels and prevent an estrogen imbalance.

Manage Stress
Stress can disrupt the body's natural hormone balance, so it is important to manage stress through techniques such as meditation, yoga, or deep breathing exercises.

Avoid Smoking And Excessive Alcohol Consumption
Smoking and excessive alcohol consumption can disrupt the body's natural hormone balance and increase the risk of an estrogen imbalance.

CHAPTER 4

Signs And Symptoms Of Estrogen Imbalance: How To Recognize Hormonal Disruption

When there is an imbalance in estrogen levels, it can cause a range of symptoms that can be disruptive to your daily life. This chapter will discuss the signs and symptoms of estrogen imbalance and how to recognize hormonal disruption.

Signs And Symptoms Of Estrogen Imbalance

Irregular Menstrual Cycle
The menstrual cycle is regulated by the balance of hormones in the body, and estrogen is one of the main hormones responsible for this. When there is an imbalance in estrogen levels, it can lead to irregular periods. This may include a

cycle that is shorter or longer than normal, spotting between periods, or missed periods.

Hot Flashes And Night Sweats

Hot flashes and night sweats are common symptoms of menopause, which is a time when estrogen levels naturally decrease. However, these symptoms can also occur when there is an imbalance in estrogen levels, even before menopause. Hot flashes are sudden feelings of warmth that can cause sweating and flushing of the skin. Night sweats are hot flashes that occur during sleep, causing you to wake up feeling hot and sweaty.

Mood Swings

Estrogen plays a role in regulating mood, and when there is an imbalance in estrogen levels, it can cause mood swings. You may feel irritable, anxious, or depressed. You may also experience mood swings that range from high to low, making it difficult to maintain a stable emotional state.

Fatigue

Fatigue is a common symptom of estrogen imbalance, especially when levels are low. You may feel tired and lethargic, even after getting enough sleep. You may also have difficulty concentrating and completing tasks.

Weight Gain

Estrogen imbalance can also cause weight gain, especially in the abdominal area. This is because estrogen plays a role in regulating metabolism and fat distribution. When there is an imbalance in estrogen levels, it can lead to increased fat storage in the abdominal area.

Vaginal Dryness

Estrogen is responsible for maintaining vaginal health, including lubrication. When there is an imbalance in estrogen levels, it can cause vaginal dryness, which can lead to discomfort during sex and an increased risk of vaginal infections.

Hair Loss

Estrogen plays a role in promoting hair growth, and when there is an imbalance in estrogen levels, it can lead to hair loss. It's possible that you've observed an increased amount of hair loss or thinning of your hair.

How To Recognize Hormonal Disruption

If you are experiencing any of the symptoms of estrogen imbalance, it may be a sign of hormonal disruption. To recognize hormonal disruption, it is important to pay attention to your body and any changes that may be occurring. Here are some tips to help you recognize hormonal disruption:

Keep Track Of Your Menstrual Cycle: If you notice changes in your menstrual cycle, such as irregular periods or spotting between periods, it may be a sign of hormonal disruption.

Pay Attention To Your Mood: If you are experiencing mood swings or feelings of depression or anxiety, it may be a sign of hormonal disruption.

Monitor Your Energy Levels: If you are feeling fatigued or having difficulty concentrating, it may be a sign of hormonal disruption.

Keep Track Of Any Changes In Weight Or Body Composition: If you are gaining weight, especially in the abdominal area, it may be a sign of hormonal disruption.

Pay Attention To Changes In Your Hair Or Skin: If you are experiencing hair loss or changes in your skin, such as acne or dryness, it may be a sign of hormonal disruption.

Should you experience any of these symptoms, do not hesitate to speak with your healthcare provider. They can perform tests to determine if there is an imbalance in your estrogen levels and recommend treatment options to help restore hormonal balance.

Treatment Options For Estrogen Imbalance

The treatment options for estrogen imbalance depend on the underlying cause and severity of the imbalance. Some common treatment options include:

Hormone Replacement Therapy (HRT): This is a common treatment option for women experiencing menopause or low estrogen levels. HRT involves taking medications that contain estrogen to help balance hormone levels.

Lifestyle Changes: Making lifestyle changes, such as eating a healthy diet, exercising regularly, and reducing stress, can help promote hormonal balance and alleviate symptoms.

Medications: There are several medications available that can help regulate estrogen levels, such as birth control pills or medications that reduce the production of estrogen.

Alternative Therapies: Some women may find relief from estrogen imbalance symptoms through alternative therapies, such as acupuncture, herbal supplements, or meditation.

It is important to discuss all treatment options with your healthcare provider to determine the best course of action for your individual needs.

CHAPTER 5

Diagnostic Testing For Estrogen Imbalance: Methods And Limitations

When the levels of estrogen are imbalanced, it can cause various health problems, including menstrual irregularities, fertility issues, osteoporosis, and breast cancer. Therefore, it is crucial to diagnose estrogen imbalance promptly to prevent and manage these conditions effectively.

Diagnostic testing for estrogen imbalance involves several methods, including blood tests, urine tests, and saliva tests. Each method has its limitations, and understanding them is essential in interpreting the results accurately. In this chapter, we will discuss the methods and limitations of diagnostic testing for estrogen imbalance.

Blood Tests

Blood tests are the most commonly used method for diagnosing estrogen imbalance. The test measures the levels of estradiol, which is the most potent form of estrogen, in the blood. Estradiol levels fluctuate throughout the menstrual cycle, with the highest levels occurring during ovulation.

Blood tests can be performed at any time during the menstrual cycle. However, the results may vary depending on the timing of the test. For instance, if the test is performed during the follicular phase, which is the first half of the menstrual cycle, the estradiol levels may be low. In contrast, if the test is performed during the luteal phase, which is the second half of the menstrual cycle, the estradiol levels may be high.

Blood tests have some limitations in diagnosing estrogen imbalance. First, they only measure estradiol levels and not other forms of estrogen, such as estrone and estriol. Second, they cannot measure the amount of estrogen that is biologically active in the body. Finally, blood tests are not accurate in diagnosing estrogen imbalance in women who are taking hormonal contraceptives, as the levels of estradiol may be artificially suppressed.

Urine Tests

Urine tests can also be used to diagnose estrogen imbalance. The test measures the levels of estrogen metabolites in the urine. Estrogen metabolites are the byproducts of estrogen metabolism, and their levels reflect the amount of estrogen that has been metabolized in the body.

Urine tests can provide a more comprehensive picture of estrogen metabolism than blood tests.

For instance, they can measure the levels of estrone and estriol, in addition to estradiol. Urine tests can also indicate the amount of estrogen that is biologically active in the body.

Urine tests can be performed at any time during the menstrual cycle. However, like blood tests, the results may vary depending on the timing of the test. For instance, if the test is performed during the follicular phase, the levels of estrogen metabolites may be low. In contrast, if the test is performed during the luteal phase, the levels of estrogen metabolites may be high.

Urine tests also have some limitations in diagnosing estrogen imbalance. First, the levels of estrogen metabolites in the urine may be affected by various factors, such as diet, medication, and environmental toxins. Therefore, interpreting the results may require specialized knowledge and experience. Second, urine tests are not accurate in diagnosing estrogen imbalance in women who are taking hormonal contraceptives, as the levels of estrogen metabolites may be artificially suppressed.

Saliva Tests

Saliva tests can also be used to diagnose estrogen imbalance. The test measures the levels of free, biologically active estrogen in the saliva. Free estrogen is the portion of estrogen that is not bound to proteins and can freely move into cells and tissues.

Saliva tests can provide a more accurate measure of biologically active estrogen levels than blood or urine tests. This is because free estrogen is the form of estrogen that exerts the most significant physiological effects in the body. Saliva tests can also measure the levels of other hormones, such as progesterone and testosterone, which are involved in the menstrual cycle and reproductive health.

Saliva tests can be performed at any time during the menstrual cycle. However, the results may vary depending on the timing of the test, similar to blood and urine tests. Saliva tests are noninvasive and easy to perform, and they can be done at home using a saliva collection kit.

Saliva tests also have some limitations in diagnosing estrogen imbalance. First, the levels of free estrogen in the saliva may be affected by various factors, such as stress and medications, which may influence the permeability of the saliva glands. Therefore, interpreting the results may require specialized knowledge and experience. Second, saliva tests are not accurate in diagnosing estrogen imbalance in women who are taking hormonal contraceptives, as the levels of free estrogen may be artificially suppressed.

Consulting with a healthcare provider who specializes in women's health is essential in interpreting the results of diagnostic testing for estrogen imbalance. They can help determine the most appropriate method for testing and interpret the results accurately. By detecting and managing estrogen imbalance promptly, women can maintain optimal reproductive and overall health.

CHAPTER 6

Treating Estrogen Imbalance: Lifestyle Changes, Medications, And Alternative Therapies

Estrogen is a hormone responsible for the development and regulation of the female reproductive system, as well as the health of bones and cardiovascular health. When estrogen levels are too high or too low, it can lead to a variety of health problems. Estrogen imbalance can affect women of all ages and can result from various factors such as stress, poor diet, medication, environmental factors, or underlying medical conditions.

We will explore the various ways to treat estrogen imbalance through lifestyle changes, medications, and alternative therapies.

Lifestyle Changes:

Lifestyle changes are often the first line of treatment for estrogen imbalance. The following lifestyle changes can help to balance estrogen levels naturally:

Exercise: Regular physical activity is beneficial for overall health and can help to regulate hormone levels. Exercise can reduce estrogen levels in women who have higher levels of estrogen and increase estrogen levels in women who have lower levels.

Balanced Diet: A healthy and balanced diet can help to regulate estrogen levels. A diet that is rich in fruits, vegetables, whole grains, lean protein, and healthy fats can help to maintain estrogen balance.

Stress Management: High levels of stress can lead to hormonal imbalances. Therefore, it is essential to manage stress levels through activities such as meditation, yoga, or deep breathing exercises.

Reduce Exposure To Environmental Toxins:
Environmental toxins such as pesticides, plastics, and synthetic hormones can disrupt the body's hormonal balance. To minimize exposure, it is best to eat organic foods, avoid using plastic containers for food storage, and use natural cleaning products.

Medications:
When lifestyle changes are not enough to balance estrogen levels, medications can be prescribed by a healthcare professional. The following medications are commonly used to treat estrogen imbalance:

Hormone Replacement Therapy (HRT): HRT is a type of medication used to supplement estrogen and progesterone levels in women who are experiencing menopause or have had a hysterectomy. HRT is available in the form of pills, patches, gels, and creams.

Birth Control Pills: Birth control pills contain synthetic estrogen and progesterone, which can regulate hormone levels and reduce symptoms of estrogen imbalance.

Aromatase Inhibitors: Aromatase inhibitors are a type of medication that can lower estrogen levels in postmenopausal women with estrogen receptor-positive breast cancer.

Alternative Therapies:
In addition to lifestyle changes and medication, alternative therapies can also help to balance estrogen levels naturally. The following alternative therapies are commonly used to treat estrogen imbalance:

Herbal Remedies: Several herbs such as Black cohosh, Red clover, and Dong quai can help to regulate estrogen levels naturally.

Acupuncture: Acupuncture is an ancient Chinese therapy that involves the insertion of needles into specific points in the body. It is believed to stimulate the body's natural healing process and can help to balance hormone levels.

Chiropractic: Chiropractic is a complementary therapy that involves the manipulation of the spine to improve health and wellness. Chiropractic treatment can help to reduce stress, improve nerve function, and balance hormone levels.

CHAPTER 7

Managing Menopause - Addressing Estrogen Imbalance and Aging

Menopause is a natural process that every woman experiences as she ages, indicating the end of reproductive years by the permanent cessation of menstrual periods. Typically occurring between the ages of 45 to 55, with an average age of 51, menopause brings a decrease in estrogen production, resulting in various physical and emotional symptoms. This chapter delves into the role of estrogen imbalance in menopause and suggests ways to manage its effects.

What Happens During Menopause?

The decrease in estrogen production during menopause results in several physical and emotional symptoms as the body undergoes changes that are a natural part of the aging process. The physical symptoms include hot flashes, night sweats, vaginal dryness, and difficulty sleeping, along with joint pain, headaches, and fatigue. Emotional symptoms may include mood swings, irritability, and depression.

Estrogen Imbalance and Menopause

A decrease in estrogen production during menopause can cause an estrogen imbalance that leads to several symptoms, including hot flashes, night sweats, vaginal dryness, and difficulty sleeping. The imbalance can also lead to an increased risk of osteoporosis, which results from the loss of bone density due to a decline in estrogen levels. Additionally, estrogen imbalance can impact cholesterol levels, increasing the risk of heart disease, as estrogen protects the heart, and a reduction in estrogen production can raise LDL cholesterol levels.

Managing Menopause Symptoms

There are different ways to manage menopause symptoms, including lifestyle changes, medications, and hormone replacement therapy (HRT).

Lifestyle Changes
Lifestyle changes can help alleviate some menopause symptoms. Eating a healthy diet, regular exercise, and avoiding caffeine and alcohol can reduce the frequency and severity of hot flashes. Wearing lightweight clothing and using a fan can help keep cool during hot flashes. Over-the-counter vaginal moisturizers and lubricants can relieve vaginal dryness. Regular exercise can also help maintain bone density, reducing the risk of osteoporosis.

Medications

Several medications are available to treat menopause symptoms. Low-dose antidepressants can reduce hot flashes' frequency and severity, while hormone therapy (HT) can alleviate physical symptoms, such as hot flashes, vaginal dryness, and joint pain. HT involves taking estrogen and progesterone to replace the hormones the body no longer produces.

Hormone Replacement Therapy (HRT)

HRT is a medical treatment that can help manage menopause symptoms by providing estrogen and progesterone. HRT comes in several forms, including pills, patches, creams, and vaginal rings. It can alleviate many physical symptoms of menopause, reduce the risk of osteoporosis, and potentially lower the risk of heart disease.

In conclusion, while menopause is a natural process, estrogen imbalance can cause physical and emotional symptoms, leading to several complications. By adopting lifestyle changes, medications, and HRT, women can manage menopause symptoms and improve their quality of life.

CHAPTER 8

Estrogen And Women's Health: The Link To Breast Cancer, Heart Disease, And Other Conditions

Unfortunately, estrogen can also increase the risk of certain health conditions, including breast cancer, heart disease, and other medical conditions. In this chapter, we will explore the link between estrogen and women's health and the associated conditions.

Breast Cancer

Breast cancer is the second most common cancer among women worldwide, and estrogen is one of the leading risk factors. Estrogen promotes the growth and development of breast tissue, and the prolonged exposure of breast tissue to high levels of estrogen can increase the risk of breast cancer. Estrogen can promote breast cell proliferation, which can lead to the development of abnormal cells that can potentially become cancerous.

Estrogen can also increase the risk of breast cancer by promoting the growth of blood vessels that supply the cancer cells with nutrients and oxygen. This process is known as angiogenesis and can facilitate the spread of cancer cells to other parts of the body.

Several factors can affect the risk of breast cancer, including age, family history, and lifestyle factors such as alcohol consumption, smoking, and physical activity. However, the role of estrogen in breast cancer risk cannot be overlooked.

Heart Disease
In the United States, women's primary cause of death is heart disease. Estrogen plays a complex role in heart health, and the impact of estrogen on cardiovascular health is not yet fully understood. Estrogen has been shown to have a protective effect on the heart, especially in

premenopausal women. Estrogen can reduce LDL (bad) cholesterol levels, increase HDL (good) cholesterol levels, and improve blood vessel function.

However, the protective effect of estrogen on the heart declines after menopause when estrogen levels drop. Postmenopausal women are at increased risk of developing heart disease, and hormone replacement therapy (HRT) has been used to manage this risk. HRT involves the use of estrogen and other hormones to alleviate the symptoms of menopause and reduce the risk of heart disease. However, HRT has been associated with an increased risk of certain medical conditions, such as breast cancer and stroke.

Other Medical Conditions
Estrogen plays a vital role in several other areas of women's health. Low levels of estrogen can lead to medical conditions such as osteoporosis, vaginal dryness, and urinary incontinence.

Estrogen replacement therapy can alleviate these symptoms and improve quality of life.

Estrogen can also affect mood and cognitive function. Low levels of estrogen can lead to mood swings, irritability, and depression. Estrogen replacement therapy can alleviate these symptoms and improve cognitive function.

However, estrogen replacement therapy is not without risks. Estrogen replacement therapy has been associated with an increased risk of stroke, blood clots, and breast cancer. Therefore, it is essential to weigh the benefits and risks of estrogen replacement therapy before starting treatment.

CHAPTER 9

Balancing Estrogen Naturally: Strategies for Optimal Hormonal Health

In this chapter, we will explore some strategies for balancing estrogen naturally to promote optimal hormonal health.

Maintain A Healthy Weight
Maintaining a healthy weight is essential for balancing estrogen levels in the body. Excess weight can lead to an increase in estrogen production, which can disrupt the balance of hormones in the body. This disruption can lead to a variety of health issues, including an increased risk of breast cancer. To maintain a healthy weight, it is essential to eat a healthy, balanced diet and engage in regular exercise.

Consume A Balanced Diet

Eating a balanced diet is essential for maintaining optimal hormonal health. A diet that is high in fruits, vegetables, whole grains, and lean protein can help to balance estrogen levels in the body. Foods that are rich in phytoestrogens, such as soy products, can also help to balance estrogen levels. However, it is important to note that excessive consumption of soy products can lead to an increase in estrogen levels, which can disrupt the balance of hormones in the body.

Reduce Stress

Stress can disrupt the balance of hormones in the body, including estrogen levels. Chronic stress can lead to an increase in cortisol production, which can interfere with the production and regulation of estrogen in the body. To reduce stress, it is important to engage in stress-reducing activities, such as meditation, yoga, or deep breathing exercises.

Get Enough Sleep

Getting enough sleep is essential for maintaining optimal hormonal health. Sleep is a critical time for the body to regulate hormone levels, including estrogen levels. Lack of sleep can disrupt this balance, leading to an increase in estrogen levels. To promote optimal hormonal health, it is essential to get at least seven to eight hours of sleep per night.

Engage in Regular Exercise

Engaging in regular exercise is essential for maintaining optimal hormonal health. Exercise can help to balance estrogen levels in the body by reducing excess weight, increasing muscle mass, and promoting a healthy circulatory system. It is recommended to engage in at least 30 minutes of moderate-intensity exercise per day to promote optimal hormonal health.

Reduce Exposure To Environmental Estrogens

Environmental estrogens are substances that mimic the effects of estrogen in the body and can disrupt the balance of hormones. These substances are found in many household products, including plastic containers, pesticides, and cleaning products. To reduce exposure to environmental estrogens, it is important to use natural cleaning products, avoid using plastic containers to store food and beverages, and choose organic foods whenever possible.

Consider Herbal Supplements

Herbal supplements can be a natural way to balance estrogen levels in the body. Supplements such as black cohosh, dong quai, and red clover have been shown to have estrogenic effects in the body, helping to balance estrogen levels. However, it is important to note that herbal supplements can have side effects and should only be taken under the guidance of a healthcare provider.

CHAPTER 10

Living With Estrogen Imbalance: Coping With The Emotional And Physical Challenges

Living with estrogen imbalance can be emotionally challenging, especially if the symptoms are severe or interfere with daily activities. Here are some tips on coping with the emotional challenges of estrogen imbalance:

Practice Self-Care: It is crucial to take care of yourself during this time. Try to get enough sleep, eat a healthy diet, exercise regularly, and engage in activities that bring you joy and relaxation.

Seek Support: Talking to friends, family members, or a therapist can help you manage the emotional stress that comes with estrogen imbalance. It's important to have a support system that understands what you're going through.

Practice Mindfulness: Mindfulness meditation or deep breathing exercises can help reduce stress and anxiety. These techniques can help you stay calm and centered during challenging times.

Take Breaks: Taking breaks throughout the day can help you manage your energy levels and prevent burnout. Take a walk outside, read a book, or listen to music during breaks.

Stay Positive: Try to focus on the positive aspects of your life and be kind to yourself. Remember that estrogen imbalance is a temporary condition, and with the right treatment and support, you can manage your symptoms effectively.

Coping With The Physical Challenges Of Estrogen Imbalance

The physical symptoms of estrogen imbalance can be uncomfortable and affect your daily life. Here are some tips on coping with the physical challenges of estrogen imbalance:

Talk to Your Doctor: If you're experiencing physical symptoms such as hot flashes or heavy bleeding, talk to your doctor about treatment options. Your doctor may recommend hormone therapy, medications, or other treatments to help manage your symptoms.

Exercise: Regular exercise can help you maintain a healthy weight, reduce joint pain, and boost your energy levels. Try to incorporate low-impact exercises such as walking, swimming, or yoga into your daily routine.

Eat A Balanced Diet: Eating a balanced diet that includes plenty of fruits, vegetables, whole grains, and lean protein can help you manage your weight and improve your overall health.

Minimize your consumption of processed foods as well as foods that are high in sugar and saturated fat.

Practice Good Sleep Hygiene: Getting enough sleep is essential for managing your symptoms. Practice good sleep hygiene by sticking to a regular sleep schedule, avoiding caffeine and alcohol before bedtime, and creating a relaxing sleep environment.

Manage Stress: Stress can worsen physical symptoms such as headaches and joint pain. Discovering healthy techniques for handling stress, such as engaging in meditation, or performing deep breathing exercises, can be beneficial.

Stay Hydrated: Drinking plenty of water can help alleviate symptoms such as hot flashes and dry skin. Experts suggest consuming a minimum of eight glasses of water daily.

Talk To A Nutritionist: A nutritionist can help you create a healthy meal plan that meets your unique needs and helps manage your symptoms.

Treatment Options For Estrogen Imbalance
Treatment for estrogen imbalance depends on the cause and severity of the condition. In some cases, lifestyle changes such as exercise, diet, and stress management techniques may be enough to manage symptoms. In other cases, medication or hormone therapy may be necessary.

Hormone therapy involves taking estrogen in the form of pills, patches, creams, or vaginal rings. Hormone therapy can help relieve symptoms such as hot flashes, vaginal dryness, and mood swings. However, hormone therapy may also increase the risk of certain health conditions such as breast cancer, stroke, and blood clots.

Medications such as antidepressants and anti-anxiety drugs may also be used to manage emotional symptoms associated with estrogen imbalance. Other medications may be used to treat specific conditions such as thyroid disorders or PCOS.

CONCLUSION

The human body is a complex and intricate machine, and when it comes to hormones, it is no exception. Hormonal imbalances are a common problem that can affect both men and women, but women are particularly vulnerable due to the cyclical nature of their hormone fluctuations. In this book, we have discussed the estrogen cycle, its impact on women's health, and how to overcome hormonal imbalances and regain vitality.

Firstly, we explored the basics of the estrogen cycle, including its various phases and how it affects the body. We learned that estrogen plays a crucial role in many bodily functions, including bone density, cardiovascular health, and reproductive health. However, too much or too little estrogen can lead to hormonal imbalances and various health problems.

Next, we delved into the impact of hormonal imbalances on women's health. We learned that hormonal imbalances can cause a range of symptoms, including mood swings, weight gain, irregular periods, infertility, and more. We also explored the links between hormonal imbalances and various health conditions, such as PCOS, endometriosis, and breast cancer.

Fortunately, we also discussed ways to overcome hormonal imbalances and regain vitality. We learned that lifestyle changes, such as a healthy diet, regular exercise, stress management, and good sleep habits, can go a long way in balancing hormones. We also explored various natural remedies, such as herbal supplements, essential oils, and acupuncture, that can help alleviate hormonal imbalances.

Additionally, we discussed conventional medical treatments for hormonal imbalances, including hormone replacement therapy, birth control pills, and other medications. We explored the pros and cons of these treatments and when they might be appropriate.

Overall, Breaking the Estrogen Cycle is a comprehensive guide to understanding hormonal imbalances and their impact on women's health. By exploring the estrogen cycle and various treatment options, we hope to empower women to take control of their health and regain vitality. It is important to note that every woman's hormonal journey is unique, and what works for one woman may not work for another. Therefore, we encourage women to work closely with their healthcare providers to find the best treatment options for their individual needs.

In conclusion, we believe that knowledge is power when it comes to hormonal imbalances. By understanding the estrogen cycle and how to overcome hormonal imbalances, women can take charge of their health and achieve optimal well-being. We hope that this book serves as a valuable resource for women everywhere who are seeking to break the estrogen cycle and regain their vitality.

Printed in Dunstable, United Kingdom